T0197323

A Conduit

Diary of an Emergency Department Chaplain

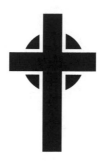

THOMAS C. TUCKER, PH.D.

WESTBOW
PRESS®
A DIVISION OF THOMAS NELSON
& ZONDERVAN

WestBow Press books may be ordered through booksellers or by contacting:

WestBow Press
A Division of Thomas Nelson & Zondervan
1663 Liberty Drive
Bloomington, IN 47403
www.westbowpress.com
844-714-3454

ISBN: 978-1-6642-2666-1 (sc)
ISBN: 978-1-6642-2667-8 (hc)
ISBN: 978-1-6642-2665-4 (e)

Library of Congress Control Number: 2021904509

Print information available on the last page.

WestBow Press rev. date: 03/16/2021

Contents

Part II 21

Teamwork: Cases That Define

My Integration into the Hospital Staff

Part III 41

Final Service: Cases for Families at
the End of Life for a Dear One

Part IV 67

Ecumenical: Cases That Serve Those
in Need without Discrimination

Part V..83

Care and Comfort: Cases That Combine
Compassion with Spiritual Care

Preface

A highly respected colleague suggested at a seminar that chaplains should write books about their experiences. I chose to adapt the form of excerpts from my memories as a start and then periodically add entries of the more remarkable events from my service to patients, their families, and the entire medical staff.

As I approach the hospital, I empty my personal thoughts and clear my focus so I can leave me outside and become a conduit, letting God's love, grace, and healing flow through me. Training and experience are important, but these are best applied by letting God direct the spiritual care provided.

My personal style of chaplaincy in a large regional emergency department with four sections and certified for trauma level II is ecumenical and eclectic. (Note: emergency department (ED) is the current term replacing emergency room (ER), which now refers to smaller hospitals and neighborhood clinics.) Timeliness is the principal characteristic, timeliness of both spiritual care and physical comfort care without impeding medical care. Staff support and teamwork with the entire medical team rounds out the principal functions.

All cases are unexpected; nobody plans a visit to the emergency department, certainly not those arriving by EMS ambulance. There is a certain level of trauma in every case; otherwise, they (patients and family) would not be in an emergency department. However, the care level *trauma* is for the most severe life-threatening cases. Health care procedures, both standard and contingency, are well defined. The staff is skilled at triage and diagnosis. As emergency department chaplain, I am challenged to identify spiritual needs at sight and be alert to diagnostic clues and pertinent information that should be shared with the medical team. Confidentiality must be maintained unless there is a threat to the patient or any other person.

Teamwork, teamwork, teamwork. The staff call me "Dr. Tom." It is both professional and friendly. Of course, the physicians are a bit more formal and call me "Dr. Tucker" as a matter of professional courtesy. They do inquire about my doctorate and are surprised to hear it is in business administration with emphasis on quantitative methods (statistics) and a minor in hospital administration. Then they smile when they learn I was a specialty hospital administrator who retired, received seminary training, and came back as a volunteer chaplain.

Here is the clincher: being an ED chaplain was not my idea. I was assigned to the emergency department by hospital administration. Within a month, I was asked to add NICU and eventually to take calls throughout the hospital, including seven ICUs. What follows may have clues as to why God chose to have this conduit placed in this fast-paced environment.

Introduction

Jesus traveled all around the Sea of Galilee and down to Jerusalem, preaching, teaching, and healing. This is a small area by today's standards, but it was a large area in His time. He traveled by foot mostly, with an occasional boat ride. He attracted all levels of society and served all who were in need regardless of their status.

My service as a chaplain is modeled after several scriptures. Look at Mark 2:1–12 as a start. Jesus, the popular miracle worker, had returned to Capernaum. He was at home, but He was preaching and teaching, not resting. The local populous flocked to His house, filled it, and overflowed out the door.

A group of people had faith Jesus could cure a paralytic. Four members of this group carried the paralytic. Pause. Who is this group, and who is carrying the paralytic? I have been assured the Greek pronoun the author of Mark used for who was carrying the paralytic is gender neutral. So, we don't know if these were men or women, boys or girls, young or old, rich or poor, Jews or Gentiles. All we know is there were more than four, they had compassion, and they were committed to getting the paralytic to Jesus.

They found they were blocked, frozen out. So many people were crowding around to hear Jesus this group could not even get close to the front door. They thought outside the box. They hauled the paralytic to the roof, broke out the shovels, and dug through the roof.

When Jesus looked up to see a hole in the roof and a paralytic being lowered, He knew what was going on. When Jesus saw their faith, He forgave the paralytic his sins, meaning He cured the paralytic. Note: Jesus saw the faith of the group—*their* faith, not that of the paralytic.

Three things stand out:

1. Compassion for the lame man
2. Action to seek help
3. Faith resulting in healing

Think about these three in your life.

This same story appears in Luke 5 and Matthew 9. The account in Matthew is then followed by a series of stories. Look at Matthew 9:18–31 next. A religious ruler had faith that Jesus could raise his daughter. On his way to the leader's house, the woman with a bleeding problem was healed. She wanted to touch His cloak, but Jesus had compassion and told her, "Your faith has healed you."

Jesus continued to the ruler's house and brought his daughter up from her deathbed, healthy. Next, Jesus invited two blind men to come inside, where He restored their sight based on their faith. They were to keep it a secret, but they told everybody anyway.

We see compassion, action, and faith again and again.

And we know Christ's compassion and action extended beyond healing to all forms of human endeavor. He fed the crowds of five thousand and four thousand out of compassion. He taught out of compassion: the Sermon on the Mount, His many parables. I am particularly sensitive to the Good Samaritan lesson (Luke 10:30–37), "Go and do likewise"; and the sheep and goats lesson (Matthew 25:31–40), "Do unto the least of these." But, most importantly, Jesus taught by example.

Now look at Matthew 9:35–38. Jesus, in His compassion, went to the ill so they could be healed by their faith. Then He commissioned His disciples to go and do likewise, telling them the harvest is plentiful, but the workers are few.

Next, turn to Luke 9:1–6. Here we are told the twelve disciples are sent to serve and heal. In Luke 10:1–12, Jesus sent seventy-two of His followers to do likewise. And … here I am today—a worker in his harvest. I have the opportunity to be God's conduit for:

Compassion,
Action,
and Faith.

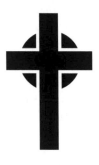

PART I

Landmarks:
Cases That Define My Service

Cases 1.1: The Call

"ACTIVE SHOOTER" scrolled across my large-screen TV early one morning. An aerial view from a helicopter showed a local high school surrounded by police cars. The reporter's voice said, "Ambulances have been seen leaving the scene." I dropped everything, grabbed my hospital jacket and credentials, jumped in the car, and headed toward the hospital, only fifteen minutes away. My hospital with its emergency department and trauma units was the nearest to the school, so I knew those ambulances were headed our way.

My phone rang as I approached the entrance to the hospital. The ED coordinator said, "Dr. Tom, can you come *now*? We need you."

I answered, "I'm already on my way. I'll be there shortly."

As I entered the hospital, a nurse recognized me and said, "We're setting up the large conference room for family and friends." It was on my way to the ED, so I stopped in.

An ED tech who was also an EMT was setting up an information table. She told everyone she was in contact with the hospital's ED and other hospitals, so she could obtain information for those trying to locate a student or teacher at the high school if they were receiving medical care.

While we had the room's attention, I prayed for the forty or so who had already assembled. I headed toward the back door of the conference room, and on the way, I stopped and prayed with a table of students who were trembling. Then I ducked out the back door into a hall that led straight to the ED.

Four trauma surgeons, their scrub nurses, and support technicians were standing by, gowned and gloved. All noncritical ED patients had been moved to other areas of the hospital. All three of the ED trauma suites were open and ready. All noncritical surgeries had been rescheduled, and the OR suites were standing by.

EMTs called in their triage assessment of the patient

they were transporting by ambulance. Highest-need patients were rolled immediately into one of the ED trauma suites for stabilization before going to the OR. Others were placed in nearby ED rooms for further assessment and stabilization. Only parents were allowed in the ER; all others were sent to the large conference room.

Eight injured students came to our ED. Two of our patients went to OR as quickly as possible. I prayed with their parents and sent them to the surgery waiting room. Two other patients had what were judged minor wounds, with bleeding controlled by bandages applied by EMTs. I was able to visit with these and their parents while the staff treated the others. When we were notified the shooter was in custody and there were no additional injured victims, the trauma surgeons who had not gone to the OR began treating wounds in the ED.

I took a break and went back to the conference room, where the crowd had tripled. The pastor from a large local church came and asked to see me. He was volunteering to work with the increasing number of family and friends who were now overflowing the large conference room. I welcomed his help, and he further volunteered to call his youth minister to work with the large number of students. I prayed with another table of students and a couple tables of family and friends and then headed back to the ED.

On the way back, a pastor friend from another denomination called me. He guessed I was in the middle of this crisis and called to pray for me. When I got back to the ED, I was able to visit with the rest of the injured students and their parents.

There was humor amid tragedy. One student was shot through the buttocks. He was lying on his stomach. He rose up on his elbows and said with a big smile, "The bullet ended up in my hip pocket."

I took a quick, light lunch break. When I returned, all the wounded students had been admitted to the hospital for observation or released to the care of their personal physician. I resumed my normal ER rounds as the patients who had been moved out temporarily were returned to the unit.

As I finished, a Catholic priest caught me in the hall. He had finished his daily calls in another hospital a few miles away. He knew I was in the ED during the crisis and came to care for me. We went to the large conference room, which was beginning to clear. We got snacks from those the hospital had provided for the large number of visitors and sat down to talk. The priest debriefed me and prayed for me.

I soaked my feet when I got home late that afternoon. As I leaned back, another pastor friend called. He knew I had been on the front line and called to pray for me. I sat back and thanked God for sending five pastors from four different denominations to support me. This is truly an ecumenical ministry.

A month later, I was recalling some of these events with a few friends. It was remarkable the number of people who came to the hospital. Two of the injured students were members of the high school baseball team, and the entire team came to the hospital. I mentioned how pleased I was that the traumatized students would let an old man talk with them, and how rewarding it was to see their faces relax from the tenseness of frozen fear. One of these friends remarked, "They needed a grandfather figure to validate their feelings and give them permission to express those feelings."

God had placed me in the right place at the right time.

Case 1.2: Attaboy #1

I entered the room and saw the patient on the bed, an elderly man sitting in the far right corner, and an elderly woman sitting diagonally opposite in the near left-hand corner. The patient was a mongoloid of advanced age, unconscious and on a ventilator.

I introduced myself and asked the patient's name. The woman explained her son was well above the life expectancy for mongoloids, and they were waiting for a feeding tube to be delivered so it could be installed surgically. She also said he never went through puberty and was still a child regardless of his size. I surmised they were going to use all life-sustaining techniques possible.

The father said he was a retired missionary who had served fifty years in the Philippines. Apparently, their son was with them that entire time. They were obviously devoted parents, and their remaining life revolved around their son. I prayed for the son and for the parents, that they would receive God's grace and that His will be done.

Both parents were weary. I offered them refreshments. They accepted coffee. I took their separate orders and returned in a couple of minutes with a fresh cup for each, with cream and sweetener as each wanted. They were quite grateful.

As I stepped out, the portable x-ray machine was wheeling by, so I stopped just outside the door to let it pass. I overheard the wife tell her husband, the former missionary, "He has a servant's heart."

That was an attaboy from God.

Case 1.3: Thank You, Jesus

The patient was a male of advanced age (I can say that, as I am of advanced age). He was lying flat, rigid as a board, staring straight up at the ceiling. His wife was sitting in a chair on the opposite wall; her head was down, and she was wringing her hands. He turned his head when I entered and immediately demanded, "Have you come to pray for me?"

I promptly replied, "Why, yes, sir. I have."

"Thank you, Jesus!" the man exclaimed. He went on to say he was a retired Baptist preacher and had been lying there praying for himself and asking if anyone was ever going to come to pray for him.

I laid hands on him and prayed for him, his wife, and the medical team. When finished, he was relaxed and serene. His wife's head was up high, and tears of joy were streaming down her cheeks.

Christ's conduit in the right place at the right time.

Case 1.4: Conduit at Work

I was walking down the main hall, headed toward the emergency department. I nodded at a man approaching and greeted him with "How are you?"

"Not so good," he replied truthfully.

I stopped cold and turned to him. He continued, "My wife is in ICU and not expected to live. I just ran home to change and get a bite to eat. We found her on the floor unconscious this morning. It's the third time in three months."

I prayed for her, for him, and for the medical team. Then I got her room number and told him I would stop by after my rounds in the ED.

It was a normal, busy day with lots of patients and families in need of spiritual and comfort care but no tragic or near-death cases. I headed up to ICU and was walking down the hall toward the room when I spotted the man and an older woman standing outside.

As I approached, he broke into a smile and introduced the woman, his mother-in-law, then said, "We just got good news. The doctor said she is going to wake up soon and will be all right. Thank you so much. This is because of you."

I felt like blushing but said, "That is good news. However, I was just God's conduit."

He replied quickly, "Then let's thank God for an effective conduit."

Case 1.5: Impromptu Funeral

I was called to visit a case that came in through the ED and was transferred to ICU. The young man was in a coma and on life support. His mother was from out of town but happened to be visiting a local friend, who accompanied her to the hospital. The mother was distraught because her son had suffered multiple strokes from blood clots thrown off by the body as it tried to fight what the doctors called "a super bug" infection that was attacking all the organs. There was no brain function left.

After prayer, I counseled her that God had many mysteries, and He would reveal them to us in His time. We often try multiple ways to deal with situations, and when none are successful, it may be God's message that we need to do something else. As we talked, she revealed more about her relationship with her son and the trials and tribulations he dealt with. She understood the gravity of the situation and appreciated the full explanations from the doctors.

As I was about to leave, she said our conversation had brought clarity to her thoughts and she understood better what lay before her. Then she asked if I could return the next day. Three of her friends who lived nearby were coming, and they all wanted to be there when she made the final decisions. I told her I would be honored to come.

I arrived the next day at the appointed time. Five

ladies were all present, the mother and her four friends. I was prepared to attend the removal of life support and be with them through the end-of-life experience. However, the mother revealed she planned to have her son cremated, and since she now lived out of state, there would be no memorial service. She asked if I would conduct a funeral at this time. She had queued two songs on her cell phone that she wanted to play during the service. I agreed.

It was an impromptu funeral. There was no obituary to read and no eulogy, and I had not prepared a message. Fortunately, I carry my pocket pastoral edition of the Book of Common Worship with me. The service consisted of lots of scripture and prayer, the mother's songs, and a few brief comments, ending with the committal. It turned out to be exactly what God had planned for this small group.

Case 1.6: Prayers Work

It was a month after a major hurricane. I stepped into the room where the patient was lying flat. As we talked, I learned he was a retired missionary to Korea.

He had fallen from a ladder doing recovery work on a house flooded by the hurricane. I prayed for God's healing grace and guidance to the medical team. He was waiting for the results of a CAT scan.

An hour later, I was passing by his room when I heard a shout: "Your prayers worked. Nothing broken." I looked in to see a broad smile and a friendly wave.

Case 1.7: Forensics

There are strict legal requirements in addition to the high standards of medical practice required of hospitals. All deaths are reported to the state through the county medical examiner. The body of a deceased patient is automatically in the custody of the medical examiner, who may release the body or hold it for examination and possible autopsy.

I reported one day just as a patient was pronounced. No family was present. I prayed for the deceased soul. As soon as the body was prepared for transportation to the morgue to be held for the ME, we heard the announcement that a gunshot victim was en route, ETA five minutes.

A nurse stripped the dirty linen, and nurses and aids began laying out equipment while I sterilized the bed. One of the nurses remarked, "Look at you," and flashed a big smile. The medical team gowned and gloved as I finished making the bed.

I stepped out to check the ambulance entrance. A

police officer was waving. I let her in. She was new and did not have the entrance code. At that time, the ambulance arrived, and I directed the EMTs to the trauma suite we had prepared. The officer stood guard at the door to the treatment room. A hospital security officer collected evidence and bagged the victim's hands while the medical team assessed and stabilized the victim.

I kept watch on the door. Two more police officers arrived and conferred with the hospital security officer on duty in the ED who made the decision to lock down the unit, as the shooter was still at large. They left to return to the scene of the shooting to assist with the investigation there, and the hospital security officer assumed duty watching the door.

My function then became visiting other patients and families, patiently and calmly, checking discretely to assure the activities associated with the shooting victim had not affected them. An hour later, I learned the rookie officer was still on duty, waiting for the detectives to come. I brought her a bottle of water.

Case 1.8: Attaboy #2

The patient was a middle-aged man who appeared to be tense and on edge. His wife was sitting beside the bed, holding her hands tightly in her lap. I greeted them, complimented the staff, and offered prayer.

As soon as I invoked God's healing grace, the muscles in his neck relaxed, and his head rested on the pillow. My prayer continued asking for comfort to his family and guidance to the medical team.

When I finished, both the patient and his wife were relaxed, and quizzical looks on their faces had been replaced with pleasantness. I offered water or coffee to his wife. He was NPO until diagnosis and a treatment plan could be determined.

As I stepped out, I heard him say to his wife, "He is an angel."

That was another attaboy from God.

Case 1.9: Made My Day

The patient and her adult son were in the room. She was nervous and apprehensive. The son was being the strong macho male. I assured her she was in the right place.

I prayed for her, her family, and the medical team. She relaxed and began to smile. They declined any comfort care, so I excused myself.

As I closed the curtain behind me, I heard the son remark, "That was the best part of my day."

And he made my day.

Cases 1.10: Ups and Downs

It was a busy day in the ED. All the rooms were full, and there were a few hall beds in use. Ambulances were arriving at the same rate as discharges. However, there were no critical cases.

I took the rare opportunity to make chaplain rounds in NICU. The census was just above average, and all the newborn infants were progressing satisfactorily. Praying for them and their families was rewarding. The parents and grandparents were delighted to have prayers of thanksgiving and for continued health and full lives. When I got home, I put my feet up and basked in the memories from NICU.

Then the call came. The victim was a teenager with a gunshot wound, and the ED staff needed help. A second call came on my way to the hospital with details of the severity of the case, ending with amazement that I was almost there.

At the hospital, I was confronted with a distraught family. The victim was on life support while doctors attempted to determine if surgery was even possible, as the bullet was embedded in the brain. The family wanted to know what happened, but police had little information themselves. In addition to spiritual care, I shepherded the family, finding a private room for them and assuring them the latest information would be promptly shared with them. Both the shock of the comatose condition of their loved one and the necessity of a forensic investigation were overwhelming.

From the heights of joy of new life being sustained to the trauma of life being ended abruptly by violence, such is the gambit of the ED chaplain.

As I was leaving, the unit clerk stopped me and said, "We so much appreciate what you do for patients, family, and staff."

I replied, "Thank you. That's the best paycheck I could get."

Cases 1.11: Present and Not Forgotten

#1. I introduced myself to the patient and offered prayer. He responded, "I called my pastor, and he has started a prayer chain. But you are here now. That's important."

#2. The next day, I entered a patient's room. She broke into a pleasant smile before I could speak. Immediately she said, "You prayed for me when I was here last year. I am so glad you are here today also."

This is the value of personal contact by an on-site hospital chaplain.

Case 1.12: Still Have Some Things to Do

There was tenseness in the room when I entered—both the elderly patient and her sons (remember, I can say elderly lovingly and knowingly). The patient said she would welcome prayer, and she added something to every phrase as I prayed, except when I prayed for healing so that she could continue to serve God and others.

When I finished, she complained she hoped God would hurry up and take her home, because she was tired of one thing after another. I suggested God may still have some things for her to do, and He wasn't going to call her home until He was ready. Almost immediately, the tension in the room lifted. Her chin lifted, and she broke into a glowing smile. Both sons widened their eyes and lifted their heads. Trust, hope, and a future returned.

Case 1.13: God's Message

When I finished praying for the elderly patient, her daughter reached out and took hold of my hand. She offered an eloquent prayer of gratitude for my service, quoting my many trips to provide nutrition, blankets, and pillows to patients and their family members. She was a retired minister and was present when I visited one of her former parishioners a few weeks before and had observed both the spiritual care and comfort care provided.

When she finished, my eyes were misty. God had sent a special message that this conduit was exactly where He wanted me to be.

Cases 1.14: Right Place, Right Time

#1. I was completing my rounds in the ED when the PA announced trauma activation. The ambulance was fifteen minutes out. I visited the last patient I had to see and went to the ambulance entrance as it pulled up. I opened the door and held up two fingers, telling the EMTs to go to trauma suite 2. They wheeled the stretcher with an accident victim straight in, without losing any time.

I brought in a blanket as the staff began cutting off the patient's clothing. I stepped to the door and was praying for the patient and staff when my phone buzzed.

#2. ICU asked me to come quickly. A complication had developed, and a patient was scheduled for immediate surgery. I slipped out the back door of ED and went down the hall to the elevator, directly to ICU. I had just a few minutes to pray with the patient and his family before the OR nurses arrived to move him to pre-op.

I stood in the hall, offering to escort the family to the surgery waiting room. They said they knew where the surgery waiting room was and were going to get something to eat and then come back.

#3. The family in the next room realized I was a chaplain and asked me to come in. The respiratory technician was there, about to remove the breathing intubation tube. The family had decided to remove life support and asked me to be with them for their father's end of life.

I prayed with them and stood by as he passed. I then conducted a brief committal service. The family expressed their appreciation and amazement. They didn't know how to contact a preacher, but I showed up anyway.

In the right place at the right time. That's how God works.

Case 1.15: All Yours

The elderly stroke victim arrived by ambulance. I visited other patients while the medical team assessed and stabilized the new arrival. An elderly man entered the unit looking lost. I asked if I could help. He said, "Room 2. They told me she is in room 2."

"Right this way, sir," I said and led him to trauma suite 2. I opened the door and let him in. X-ray, lab techs, nurses, and doctors hustled in and out.

When the flow of medical personnel slowed, I went into the room. The neurosurgeon was explaining that the patient had a severe stroke, and it was apparently twelve hours old, which meant drugs to lessen the severity were no longer effective. They could remove the blood clot to prevent further damage, but her left side would most likely remain paralyzed. The husband responded, "I don't want her to die. Go ahead."

The doctor nodded and said, "We'll prepare for surgery immediately." She turned to me, introduce herself, thanked me, and said, "All yours." She left to prepare.

I prayed for the patient, her husband, and the entire medial team. Then I accompanied them as the patient was rolled to the elevator and taken up to neurosurgery prep.

Case 1.16: Golden Feedback

The patient was a young man (probably thirty, but at my age, that is young). I offered prayer. He hesitated, pretending he had it all under control. I suggested we can never get enough prayer. He consented. When I finished, he wiped some tears. I brought him a pillow and excused myself to go to the next room.

A few minutes later, a nurse called out as we passed in the hall. "Dr. Tom." I turned. She continued, "I wanted to say thank you for praying for the patient in 18. He said that was just what he needed."

I replied, "Thank you. That is golden feedback."

PART II

Teamwork:

Cases That Define My Integration into the Hospital Staff

Case 2.1: Welcome to the Team

The attending physician, who happened to be the medical director of emergency services, and I arrived at the patient's room at the same time. I stepped aside, but the doctor said, "You first. They need you more." He knew I would address the patient's spiritual needs quickly and not delay his diagnosis and treatment.

This was my validation that I was a member of the medical team. Of course, if this were a trauma case, medical treatment would be primary, and spiritual care would be offered from the sideline for the time being.

Thomas C. Tucker, Ph.D.

Case 2.2: A Christmas Present

It was Christmas Day with low patient census and skeleton staff. I stopped by the emergency department to visit patients on this holiday, knowing none of them wanted to be in the hospital, especially on Christmas Day, and to deliver a tin of cookies for the staff.

An ambulance rolled in. The ambulance EMTs lifted an unconscious woman onto the bed in trauma suite 2. Fluids and waste fell on the floor. The associate medical director exclaimed, "On this day when we celebrate the Lord's birth, would it be too much to ask for a pair of booties to protect my new shoes?"

Staff was busy stabilizing and assessing the patient. I located the box of shoe covers, only to find it was empty. No spare staff, so I headed to the supply room, where I found a package of disposal surgical scrubs and extracted a pair of paper shoe covers. I returned and gave them to the doctor's assistant, who slipped them on the doctor's feet.

I started to leave the room, but the charge nurse called out, "We need two more, Dr. Tom." Off I went on a round trip to the supply room.

The medical staff didn't skip a beat delivering timely treatment.

Cases 2.3: Hurricane Relief

Staff is split into two groups for disaster coverage. One group is called in to stay through the disaster, and the other is on call to relieve the first group as soon as the disaster is over. Only employees and critical patients remain in the hospital during an emergency. The building is closed and secured. The emergency entrance remains open for ambulances if needed.

As soon as it was safe to travel after a major hurricane, I was able to find a restaurant that was not damaged. I loaded the back of my SUV and brought in Chinese food for the emergency staff that remained at the hospital throughout the hurricane. It was welcome relief from a steady diet of cafeteria pasta.

Two days later, a local Catholic priest and I led an ecumenical healing service for all hospital staff.

Case 2.4: Maid Service

I finished a visit with a patient and her family. As I stepped into the hall, a nurse hustled by, pushing an empty wheelchair. "Dr. Tom, can you put a sheet on 18?" she called over her shoulder.

"Certainly," I replied and went to room 18. A patient

had just been discharged from that room. Housekeeping had cleaned the room but had not made the bed. The linen cabinet in the room was empty. I went to linen supply and returned with three fitted sheets. I placed two in the empty linen cabinet in the room and began to stretch the third sheet on the bed.

The nurse returned with a patient in the wheelchair as I was pulling the final corner tight. "Thanks," she said. "This one just walked in, and we need to get her to bed quickly."

Case 2.5: Gowns

"Trauma activation, room 3," was announced over the PA. That is a cue for me to go to that trauma suite to escort any family to the family room so the medical team can focus on the patient. Family had not arrived yet. The EMTs were just rolling the patient into the room. It was an open head wound case. Nurses were gloved and putting on gowns. I grabbed a handful of paper gown packages and passed them out.

A technician dashed in and began hooking up monitoring lines. As she moved around the foot of the bed, I held up a gown. She stuck her arms straight out and walked into the gown without breaking stride. She turned her head a few seconds later and said with a big smile, "Thanks. I was so busy I forgot."

The attending physician was at the head of the bed and called for a face shield. He fit it on his head and pulled the shield down. I was about to leave when the charge nurse called out, "We need one more, Dr. Tom," and nodded at the physician.

I opened a package and held the gown for the doctor to slip on. He was a big man, and I had to lift the gown up to get it over his shoulders. His assistant tied it for him.

Later in the day, I was walking down the hall from one patient room to another when the physician approached. "Thanks for the gown. That was a big help," he said with a nod and a smile. From that day on, he smiles when he sees me on the unit.

Case 2.6: Missing Bed

I received a call from the cardiac intensive care unit requesting I visit a patient and his family. I informed the emergency department manager, who quickly said, "Go." The patient had lapsed into a coma, and the family needed spiritual care and prayer.

As I entered the back hallway on my return to the ED, I heard a PA announcement, "Immediate bed for

EMS, room 8." I rounded the corner, and there was the ambulance stretcher against the hall wall, but the patient was still on it, and the EMTs were just standing there.

I looked in room 8. No bed. Whoops. I started to look for the charge nurse when an aide appeared, pushing the bed that had been used to transport the previous patient in room 8 to another service in the hospital.

The aide wheeled the bed into the room and began to strip the used linen. No time to call housekeeping to clean the room. I grabbed a pair of gloves and a wad of disinfectant wipes and began to clean the mattress and bed rails while the aide cleaned the lines to monitoring equipment and other surfaces in the room. This allowed the nurse assigned to the new patient to receive a report from the EMTs. The aide and I made the bed while the nurse obtained information from the patient.

The EMTs moved the patient from their stretcher to the bed, and the nurse began the proper immediate care procedures. No treatment time was lost as the result of a little teamwork.

Case 2.7: Assuming Custody

I was alerted that this was a particularly tragic case. The mother had accidently smothered her newborn child.

She said she had fed the baby and fell asleep. When she woke two hours later, he was under her T-shirt not breathing. A double whammy: both grief and guilt.

Many family members filled the family room to overflowing. I introduced myself. A cousin of the mother told me they were Jehovah's Witness. I offered water and coffee and said I would be available if they had any questions.

There were two men standing outside. They had married into the family but were not Jehovah's Witness. They let me know they appreciated my presence as a spiritual caregiver.

The medical examiner would have to validate the accidental death, so the body was in the custody of the ME office. The family was informed they could view the body but not touch it. A hospital security officer was assigned custody.

A code gray was announced, which is a call for security, usually an unruly patient or family member. Regardless, the security officer had to respond. The emergency department manager came to assume custody.

Simultaneous trauma alerts arrived. The emergency department manager had to assist with case management. She turned to me. I said I would stay and assume custody.

It was time to get the body to the morgue. The cousin who was the family spokesperson was cooperative and let the family members know it was time for their final goodbyes until the funeral.

I was the second-level substitute custodian, better known as a team member.

Case 2.8: Hustling

I was called to another unit in the hospital. As I swiped my ID to open the rear door to the emergency department, the medical director and another physician were about to enter. The medical director interrupted his conversation with his colleague to reach out and shake my hand. "How are you? Good to see you," he said brightly.

I answered, "Hustling to keep up with you all."

He quickly replied, "We're hustling to keep up with you."

Case 2.9: Virgin Ears (Not)

I am on my feet, going from room to room to visit patients and their families. I do not have a workstation to sit at, so I grab a cup of coffee and go to the staff break room.

A nurse was describing a particularly demanding patient. As I sat down, she uttered a derogatory comment not usually suitable for mixed company, then immediately turned to me and said, "Oh! I'm sorry. Pretend I didn't say that."

I smiled and replied, "Hey, no problem. These are not virgin ears."

The whole room snickered.

Then a nurse I knew through another spiritual fellowship spoke up. "Oh yes, I can verify he's heard it all." Everyone continued as if I were not there.

When I finished my coffee and started to leave, another nurse said, "You need to stop in more often."

Case 2.10: Visiting Physician

I entered the room of a female patient. Her husband was present, as was another man in business shirt and tie. I stepped to the bedside when I noticed the stethoscope around the man's neck. He was a private physician, so he was not in a hospital physician's coat.

I started to back off, but he said, "I'm through. Go ahead."

I prayed for the patient, her family, and the medical staff.

As I turned to leave, the visiting physician gave me a warm smile and said, "Thank you," as he returned to the patient's bedside.

Case 2.11: Meal Service

I entered ED room 15 and found a male patient standing at the foot of his bed, straining against his monitoring cables and frantically trying to reach the paper towel dispenser. He stopped and returned to his bed, then sat on the side. I pulled out a paper towel and gave it to him.

He began to calm down and explained that his wife and his father were both receiving cancer treatments, and he was trying to care for both. He had just received his own cancer diagnosis and was scheduled for surgery in two days. The load was overwhelming, and he was having multiple secondary reactions like upset stomach and bowels.

I listened attentively and then prayed for him.

Just as I finished, a staff physician from the hospital came in. I started to leave, but he indicated for me to stay. He told the patient there was no indication of complications and that he should rest until his surgery.

The patient was relieved and leaned back on the bed. The doctor told the patient he would see what he could do about ordering a tray.

I asked if I could get a sandwich and cold drink for the patient since it was between mealtimes and the cafeteria would take a while to prepare a special tray.

The doctor smiled and said, "Absolutely." I took the patient's order and returned with it in a few minutes.

Spiritual care, teamwork, and comfort care—a winning combination.

Cases 2.12: Staff Healing

Eleven staff members valiantly gave their every skill trying to save a teenage girl.

When the family had left and the case was completed, I asked the charge nurse to assemble the staff for a debriefing. It turned into a healing service for the staff.

Patients and their families are affected, but staff is as well.

All are in need of spiritual care.

Case 2.13: Close the Door

I was taking cup of coffee to a patient. I passed by trauma suite 2, where a respiratory treatment was being administered that could be heard in the hall.

The nurse treating another patient in the room

across the hall called to me, "Dr. Tom, can you close the door?" and nodded at the trauma room. Aides rushing in and out to assist the respiratory therapist had left it open.

I closed the door, and the nurse across the hall mouthed, "Thank you."

I returned a thumps-up. There was no interruption of care for either patient with just a little teamwork, and my patient's coffee was still hot.

I later returned to the trauma room and the room across the hall to pray for the respective patients.

Cases 2.14: Follow Him

#1. A female patient was acting out both vocally and physically. I came to the commotion to offer what support I could. The patient bolted, ran to a hall bathroom, and locked herself in. The head nurse immediately used the emergency key to unlock the door. Security was called to assist with the situation.

At that instant, an ambulance arrived with an infant in distress, held by her mother on their stretcher. The route to the pediatric ED section was blocked by personnel dealing with the acting-out patient. The adult trauma suites were all occupied.

I stepped up and said I would take the EMTs by the

back route. The head nurse turned to the EMTs, said, "Follow him," and quickly returned to the crisis she was dealing with.

I led the EMTs out a side door, down a hall to the rear entrance for the pediatric ED section and used my badge to open that door. I informed the pediatric nurses the main hall was blocked temporarily. They promptly took charge of the ill infant.

What a compliment to be trusted with patient care and to assist at times of crisis.

#2. EMTs rolled the stretcher to the ED check-in desk and announced hurriedly, "ICU transfer."

The head nurse looked up, surprised, and replied, "Down the hall to the right, through the door and right again, but you'll need a badge." She looked around and mumbled, "And we're busy."

"I'll get them there," I volunteered.

"Follow him," the head nurse said. "Dr. Tom will get you there."

Off we went. I badged the direct elevator from ED to surgery and ICU and punched the ICU floor. Quick prayer on the short elevator ride. Then I led the EMTs to the assigned ICU room and headed to the ICU nursing station.

"Room 310 arriving by ambulance," I announced. The nurse on duty jumped up and hustled to the room.

When I headed back, a security guard asked, "Is it always this busy?"

"All the time," I answered.

Case 2.15: Thank You

It was an average day in the ED, with the usual wide variety of treatment and care needs. There was only one terminal case, which was transferred to ICU in preparation for organ donation. I escorted the family to the ICU waiting room and returned to the ED.

I was asked to step into the break room for a cup of coffee. I sat down to enjoy the break.

A handful of nurses talked superficially. The door opened, and the unit clerk made a beeline straight at me with a card in her hand. It was a "Thank You, Dr. Tom" card for Clergy Appreciation Day, signed by the unit manager and many of the staff.

I was overwhelmed and had to use some of my own Kleenexes. Then some of the nurses present shared stories of working with me. Those were even more touching than the card.

Case 2.16: Got You Covered

Certain patients are assigned sitters who are with the patient constantly to observe, provide minor assistance, and call for help when required. Sitters are relieved by a nursing aide for a thirty-minute lunch break. I always check with sitters (usually two or three on the unit) to see if they need anything. Occasionally, I sit in for two minutes so they can take a bathroom break when there is no other staff available.

I spotted a sitter standing at the door of a room and asked if there was anything I could do. She said she was trying to flag a nurse to get some crackers and juice for the patient.

I asked what the patient wanted. She said graham crackers and apple juice. The patient corrected to orange juice. "Got you covered," I said and took off for the patient nutrition room to return with the refreshments.

That opened the opportunity for prayer.

Teamwork opened the door for comfort care and spiritual care.

Cases 2.17: Extra Hands and Trauma Response

#1. I was passing by when I heard, "We need some extra hands here!"

I donned a pair of gloves and stepped into the room. A nurse was attempting to draw blood for diagnostic testing. Another nurse was holding the patient's shoulders and trying to keep her arm still to avoid injury. The patient's daughter was lying across her hips, trying to hold her body still. The patient squirmed, drawing her knees up and trying to buck her daughter.

I grabbed her ankles and held her legs straight. When the patient next tried to buck, she could not draw her knees, and the others were able to hold her still.

When the nurse finished, she said, "Dr. Tom, you are special."

The daughter then noticed I was a chaplain, and we had prayer.

#2. I was headed toward the next room when a nurse pushing a portable EKG said, "Dr. Tom, can you get this bed in room 7? There's a trauma alert arriving."

She next instructed an aide to get some additional equipment.

I released the brake on the empty hall bed and rolled it into room 7, which was being converted into a trauma room. I had just finished pulling the last corner on the sheet when the ambulance stretcher rolled in.

I escorted the accompanying family member to the family room for prayer while we waited for the medical team to get treatment started.

Case 2.18: No, You're Not

A hospital physician I had not met came on the unit and was about to enter the room I had just left. I introduced myself and told him I was retired.

Before I could complete my statement that I had come back as a volunteer, he said, "No, you're not. You're working as hard as anyone, and it is needed."

He followed up with a warm handshake.

It is nice to be an integral part of the medical team.

Cases 2.19: Thanks for the Info

#1. The patient seemed distraught. I offered a kind ear. She accepted prayer.

I was about to leave when her mother complained they were not getting any attention and could not find their nurse. They had been in the ED for several hours and had hardly seen anyone. She said they were about to leave. I offered a kind ear to the mother also.

The unit was busy as usual. I headed directly to the charge nurse's station and reported, "You have a dissatisfied family member in room 19, complaining of lack of care and threatening AMA (leaving against medical advice)."

The charge nurse stood immediately and said, "Thank you," then headed for room 19.

#2. I entered a room and saw the patient taking some pills from a prescription bottle in her purse.

I prayed for her and her sister who was with her. They declined comfort care, saying they were just waiting for information from the assigned nurse.

I went directly to the nursing station and reported what I had observed. All medications taken while in the hospital must be dispensed by the hospital pharmacy and properly charted for obvious reasons.

A hurried but emphatic "Thank you!" from the nurse as she headed to the room to find out what the patient had taken.

Case 2.20: I'll Return It

A bare stretcher, with no mattress, just steerable wheels, and side rails, is kept in the ambulance entrance portico. It is wheeled to the heliport for helicopter EMTs to place the flight backboard on and transport an emergency patient to a trauma suite.

One day, I spotted air ambulance attendants returning the stretcher to its location and beginning to pick up their portable equipment to make a couple of trips to the helicopter.

"Roll it out to the chopper," I said. "I'll return it."

I followed as they rolled the stretcher to the helicopter and transferred all their equipment directly while the pilot began his preflight checklist.

"Thanks so much," the flight nurse said. "That saved us a couple of trips. We're back in service sooner."

They boarded the helicopter as I wheeled the stretcher back to its standby location.

PART III

Final Service:

Cases for Families at the End of Life for a Dear One

Case 3.1: Immigrants

I was called to trauma suite 2 and informed the patient had been pronounced. His wife was in the family room by herself. She was downcast and wringing her hands.

She and her husband were from China and had work visas as medical researchers in a nearby facility. They were physicians in China. She was quite distraught that she could not save her husband from an apparent heart attack.

She shared more of their life and that in China they had no religion of any form. She was very open and receptive to spiritual care.

Their son had recently graduated from a major university and was employed near there, but it was a hundred miles away on the other side of the city, and rush hour was starting. It would take him three or four hours to get to our hospital, so he would not arrive before the body needed to be sent to the morgue for the medical examiner.

She explained the usual process in China, where all deceased are cremated, and asked about the process in our country. I explained the need for an autopsy when the deceased was not under direct care of a doctor and the cause of death had to be confirmed. Then I said that our procedure was for a funeral home to make the final arrangements with the family. That could be cremation, burial, or shipping to another location.

She was very understanding and accepted suggestions to do a Google search for a nearby funeral home. We then viewed the body for the last time.

As I was parting, she grabbed my hand and said, "I want to know more about this Christianity." I gave her the name of a Chinese church in the vicinity.

The next week, a nurse came up to me. "I was off yesterday. Sorry for the delay," she began. "The wife of the Chinese gentleman that passed last week brought this for you."

It was a thank-you note.

Case 3.2: Precious Child

I was headed toward a room in the ED with a cup of coffee for a patient and was almost run over by a nurse hurrying toward the pediatric ED area. When I stepped out of my patient's room a few moments later, I had to dodge the same nurse pushing an empty portable incubator at a speed just short of sprinting.

My curiosity led me to watch where she was going. She went directly to trauma suite 3, where an aide was removing the adult bed.

Before I could get to that room, I was blocked by the charge nurse as she grabbed a wheelchair and helped a young lady in business office attire into it. The woman was not able to stand and appeared quite distraught. A friend was trying to console her. They went toward the family room.

At that instant, the fire chief from a neighboring city burst through the ambulance entrance. "Do you have the child?" a nurse asked.

"No, they're right behind me," he answered. "I was clearing traffic."

I went to the ambulance door, and sure enough, an ambulance was rolling to a stop. I stood by as the EMTs pulled the stretcher out, then hit the button to open the doors for them, saving them a few seconds keying in the entrance code. An EMT was running beside the stretcher, using two-finger compressions on an infant. The baby was blue. I held up three fingers and pointed. They went straight to trauma suite 3.

The charge nurse returned. As she entered the trauma suite, she said to me, "The mother is not prepared for this. She's in the family room." Ah, that was the young lady.

I went to the family room, where the mother was still physically shaking. Her friend, perhaps her sister, was trying to calm her. I reached out and took her hands and got her to look at me. I explained how professionally qualified the medical staff was and that I believed whatever was going to happen was in God's hands, and he would use that staff. She calmed down. I offered a prayer.

At that time, a police officer arrived and began to take a report. The mother had just returned to work after maternity leave, and the child was in day care. The infant was found unresponsive, and EMS had been called.

As it happened, a police lieutenant was in the day-care facility's parking lot and heard the call. She was the first officer on the scene.

The police officer taking the report explained that they were making a full investigation and there would be one of two outcomes: harm that would result in criminal charges, or neglect that would not justify charges. Regardless, he said, all evidence would be available for civil action. The mother had some unkind words to say about the day care, and he let her vent some of her overwhelming emotions.

The ED doctor came in. There was nothing they could do. According to the police lieutenant on the scene within seconds of the call, the child was blue already. Even the EMTs were too late.

The mother collapsed. Her friend cradled her on the floor of the family room. We could only let her cry it out.

When the father came in, all she could say was, "She is gone." More sobs, and then she wailed, "She's not here anymore!" The father just stood there in shock, unable to speak, completely stunned by the sudden trauma.

Family began to arrive. Both sets of grandparents were grief-stricken. Several aunts and uncles joined, filling the family room. As the aunts and uncles were older teenagers and young adults, it appeared this was the first child of the next generation, making the tragedy even more severe. I was able to have prayer with the assembled family. Water and Kleenex were provided for all.

The family was informed they could come to the trauma suite to view the child. Mother and father declined. I escorted the paternal grandparents first, then the maternal grandparents.

I continued to encourage the mother and father to see their precious infant, as this would be their last memories of her. I knew it would help them accept her death and begin to penetrate denial. Eventually, the father and some of the aunts and uncles came to view.

Child Services from the hospital came with an infant death care package from NICU. The mother finally came to the trauma suite. She and the father sat while Child Service personnel cut locks of hair for each of them. Then both the father and mother helped as Child Services made footprints of the infant, copies of which would be placed in the care package.

This broke the stigma of touching the child. The father held her for several minutes. Finally, the mother agreed to hold her daughter for the last time.

The time came to transport the body to the morgue before natural deterioration began. Now the mother did not want to let go. I asked if she would let me personally carry her precious child to the morgue. She nodded and handed the infant to me.

I placed her in the portable incubator. Then I removed the hospital blanket in which she was wrapped and gave the blanket to the mother to keep.

The family all left. A nurse brought a child-size body bag, which was still three times too big. I placed the toe tag on the child and laid her in the body bag. I closed the bag and put another tag on the zipper. Then I folded the excess bag under and placed the body in the portable crib. I covered the crib with a blanket and wheeled it down the back hall to the morgue.

Security and administration met me at the morgue to unlock the door and log in the case. I lifted the precious child onto the adult-size tray and slid it into a holding vault. Then I placed an identifying sticker on the door of the vault. Security locked the morgue, and I returned the incubator to the pediatric section of the ED.

My final service to this beautiful child of God and her family was complete.

Case 3.3: Altered Reality

It was early afternoon on a mild summer day. "This is a tough one," the nurse said. "Teen suicide, room 4." A teenage girl had hung herself with the power cord of her computer over a door. Her younger brother found her.

The family was in the family room. The brother was remorseful. The mother was dumbstruck and in shock. The father was angry.

First things first, I thought. "Let's have prayer," I offered. In addition to my usual prayers at the time of death, I prayed for each of us to be able to accept God's mysteries and not demand answers.

Details began to unfold. She had been despondent and lackadaisical for a few days. It appeared she was mostly bored with nothing to do during the summer. She was on Facetime with a boyfriend in another state. Her brother had been with her that morning, and she appeared to be OK. So he went to take a shower. He found her when he returned. Both he and their mother lifted her and let her down before they called 911.

The father wanted to blame the boyfriend. But the brother said the boyfriend was a good guy and had tried to talk his sister out of it. He explained she had talked about suicide ideation with the boyfriend over the internet, and the boyfriend didn't like it. The brother said he did not think his sister was serious, just making idle talk. The father was perplexed.

I began to talk about acceptance—that acceptance

does not mean approval; it just means recognition of reality. I offered the suggestion that the girl was in an altered state of reality. We do not know about that type of reality; we can only accept what she did while in that state. The tension in the room dropped dramatically. Everyone began to relax.

The family's pastor arrived. He served a small Bible church. The pastor had a full-time job outside the church but left to come to the hospital.

When he heard *suicide*, he stiffened. That was a sin in his eyes, but he held his tongue. The family explained that the doctor had told them she had been without oxygen long enough to have completely ceased brain function. He seemed to focus on that rather than how oxygen had been cut off. I let it ride.

I went with him to view the body. Upon entering the room, he went to the body and demanded the demons leave, and he exhorted Jesus to restore all the damaged brain cells. I said nothing.

When he finished, I reported to him that I had worked with the family on acceptance. I had pointed out to them that acceptance does not mean approval, just recognition of reality. I mentioned that the girl had been in an altered state of reality, and we have no way of knowing what that is like. All we can do is accept it.

About that time, the family came in. The pastor turned to them and pronounced that she was in an altered state of reality and we could not judge her because we were not able to understand that state.

I excused myself. My job there was done.

Case 3.4: Stages of Grief

What was a high school freshman who had made the varsity softball team doing lying under a sheet in the ED? Only the medical examiner could answer that question. This was a star athlete—intelligent, healthy, and well developed. Her mother found her unresponsive when she attempted to wake her daughter for school that morning.

I prayed with the family, asking for comfort and acceptance of His divine will and giving thanks for the promise of eternal life. Then we went to the room to see this young girl.

The mother berated herself. She said she let her daughter sleep in fifteen minutes extra that day, and if she had gone to wake her at the regular time, she could have saved her. Not difficult to recognize this as the classic grief stage of blame.

The father stood there and pleaded with God to take

him instead. He said he had a bad heart, so he wanted to trade places with her. Not difficult to recognize this as the classic grief stage of trading.

The older brother stood there looking at her. He remarked that he saw her and knew she was not alive, but he did not know what that meant. Not difficult to recognize this as the classic grief stage of denial.

We returned to the family room. After additional prayer, I counseled them to seek grief counseling, as this sudden traumatic event would be with them for some time, but with God's help and the support of others, they would work through it. At this time, they could only just begin to understand the magnitude of that task.

I suggested to the nurse assigned to the case that it would be a good idea if the family gave her permission to call the school administration and alert their counseling staff so they would be prepared to work with the softball team and other students.

Case 3.5: Letting Go

The nurse said, "Dr. Tom, the family is in the family room, but the mother will not join them. She is at the bedside in trauma suite 2."

After prayer with the family, I invited them to view

the departed, but they replied they wanted to stay in the family room. I went to the trauma suite.

The mother was sitting at the side of the bed, holding the hand of her young adult daughter. She had been intubated, but the medical team was unable to resuscitate her. The mother said her daughter did not have any medical problems and she could not provide any information to help the medical team when they were attempting to save her. She neglected to mention her daughter was obese, but that was a matter for the medical examiner.

I prayed for her and for her daughter. Then she asked me to tell the family she wanted to stay with her daughter and not join the family in the family room because she wanted to be with her daughter when the medical examiner came.

As I was relaying the message to the family, the pastor from their church came. He asked me to lead another prayer for all, which I did.

The attending nurse called me aside to let me know it was time to take the body to the morgue. I returned to the family room and informed them it was time for last viewing, but they declined.

I went back to the trauma room and informed the mother it was time to take her daughter to the morgue for proper care until the medical examiner came. She looked puzzled. I told her I would personally escort her daughter to the medical examiner. She relaxed, picked up her purse, and slowly left the room. Her husband and other family members were passing by, and they joined her to leave the unit.

I reported to the charge nurse that the body could be transported to the morgue. She said the unit was terribly busy, and they needed the trauma room for new patients. I offered to be an extra pair of hands. She smiled broadly and nodded approval.

After completing preparation of the body, I assisted the attending nurse in rolling the bed down the back hall to the morgue. Security and administration met us, unlocked the door, and logged in the case.

That was when we discovered the morgue was full. Administration gave instructions, and we created a usable vault. It took three people to lift the body while I held the created tray in place.

The extra hands were needed.

Case 3.6: What Happened?

The call came in the middle of the evening. "Dr. Tom, can you come? We have an infant mortality." I responded I would be there in twenty minutes.

When I arrived, I found an infant boy on the bed and a security guard in the room. The grandfather was sitting at the side of the bed, but at the foot, not near the body. No one was to touch the body. I began to identify the situation.

The child lived with his grandparents, who reported they found him lying in the hallway and called 911. Nothing was said about how the baby got to the hallway. The mother and father were teenagers and claimed they were not in the house at the time. They were silent but not upset. Extraordinarily little else was said. I prayed for the infant and for the family in general.

Two police officers appeared. They separated the family members discretely. One of them said detectives were on their way. I surmised the death was under suspicious circumstances and that the ED doctor had promptly reported it to the authorities.

Two detectives came and began to collect statements and evidence. They said Child Services investigators were on their way. The crime scene unit had been called also but would go to the house first.

Two plainclothes female officers with Children Services ID badges arrived. They asked where they could hold private interviews with the parties. As usual, the ED was busy, so I could not confiscate a patient room. However, the family room was available. It was at the other end of the emergency department, but the officers said that was even better.

I informed the charge nurse. She said absolutely and thanked me for solving the problem for her.

Case 3.7: Not Alone

EMS called to report they were transporting a car-truck accident victim with severe injuries. The case was identified as a *trauma activation*, meaning be ready for anything. (*Trauma alert* is code to stand by for triage to determine severity.)

Several firemen in their coats and boots were in the ambulance and assisted the EMTs in unloading the stretcher. The EMT making the report said the victim was crushed under a cement truck that had turned over onto his car. Apparently, the Jaws of Life had been used to extract the victim.

The ED doctor pronounced the patient soon after arrival. Within minutes, police officers were in the room getting information for their traffic death report. I provided paper bags for them to collect what evidence they required.

I asked one of the EMTs if there was any family

THOMAS C. TUCKER, PH.D.

coming. He said, "No, the poor guy died alone. Police have not yet notified the family." That meant a police chaplain would accompany an officer to make the notification.

I responded, "He's not alone now. I will be with him until we transport him to the morgue."

Case 3.8: Vital Information

The patient arrived by ambulance with a report that he had been throwing up blood. The family followed the ambulance. I escorted them to the family room while the medical team assessed, started IVs, including transfusion, and attempted to stabilize the patient.

The wife, daughter, and a friend were all distraught. I acknowledged their concern and the suddenness of this and offered a prayer.

I then asked about their experience as an entry to ventilating the accumulating emotions. The daughter offered that she was a nurse at one of the neighborhood urgent care clinics, and she was concerned about the amount of blood. I acknowledged her account as she described it.

I inquired how it started. She said her father had stage 4 lung cancer and was undergoing treatment. He had felt fine the day before and that morning as well. They were enjoying breakfast when he began projectile vomiting blood.

I excused myself as quickly as possible and reported the daughter's information directly to the charge nurse. She stopped what she was doing and went directly to the trauma suite to relay it to the attending physician. It was vital information that had not been previously reported.

I returned to the family room. The doctor came in a short while later and reported they were unable to get a pulse. He suspected a lung tumor had eaten into a major vessel.

The daughter asked, "And that caused him to bleed out?" The physician nodded.

I stayed with the family and prayed with them. They began to make phone calls to notify other family and friends. Then I accompanied them to the bedside to view their loved one.

Case 3.9: Enough

I was informed there was a trauma activation case in trauma suite 2 and the family was in the family room. I peeked in the trauma suite, saw CPR being administered to a female, and then went to the family room.

The husband, two adult children, and their spouses were already in the family room. They were nervous and upset. I prayed with them, then brought water and coffee.

The attending nurse came to inform the family that the patient had been revived and was being stabilized. Then the nurse asked for her medical history and the current circumstances that brought on the attack. The husband then began to try to call his wife's brothers and sisters.

I went back to check on the patient. CPR was being administered a second time. I knew I would need to remain with the family while the crisis continued.

The physician invited the husband to come to the treatment room. I went with him. The physician reported that they had performed CPR twice and were only able to get a weak pulse. The prognosis was not good. The husband asked the doctor to continue treatment because he wanted to consult with his wife's relatives before making the decision.

We returned to the family room while he continued to make calls and leave messages. He wanted to see his wife again while he waited for his calls to be returned.

I returned to the trauma suite with him. He was watching her when her heart stopped again.

CPR was started immediately. After three minutes, the aide making compressions stopped while the doctor checked for pulse. A second aide resumed CPR for another three minutes. Still no pulse. It was a nurse's turn to perform CPR. I placed a step stool at the patient's bedside for her to stand on. After three minutes, a weak pulse was restored.

The husband watched all this. The physician came over but didn't have to speak. The husband said he had not heard from the relatives yet, but he could not put her through that again; that was enough. The doctor confirmed that it was a DNR (do not resuscitate) decision. The husband said it was, and the doctor entered the order.

We returned to the family room. Ten minutes later, the doctor came in. Her heart had stopped, and she was gone.

I led another prayer with the family. In a few minutes, I accompanied them to the treatment room to view the body.

Case 3.10: Tragedy and Cooperation

The call woke me just before midnight. "Dr. Tom, we have an infant death. The family has asked for a chaplain. Can you come?"

I replied, "I'll be there within a half hour."

The father was with his deceased daughter and was severely distraught. Head trauma was evident. Several family members had come to the pediatric ED and were coming in to view the body one by one. I prayed with each one.

A police officer arrived and began to photograph the child's injuries.

The story began to unfold. The couple had just had a second child. They were moving into a larger apartment. The mother came out to move the car. The toddler followed her out and went behind the car without the mother's knowing.

She had hit her own child and was being detained by police at the scene. She had the newborn with her. The father rode in the ambulance with the injured child.

The head nurse and I conferred with the police officer to see if it was possible for the mother to come to the ED to see her daughter before sending the body to the medical examiner. We explained the need to assist the mother with her grief process. The police officer communicated with the lead investigator at the scene.

Child Life Services were not in since it was past midnight. We followed hospital and legal procedures and protocol while providing counseling and comfort to the family.

Case 3.11: Honor Walk

I was called to attend end of life for an organ donor. When I arrived, the family was preparing for an honor walk. I was able to pray with the wife. When I stepped out, the Gift of Life team briefed me on their plans. I had worked with organ donation cases and knew of the coordination Gift of Life provided, but this was the first formal ceremony I had encountered.

The donor was a staff nurse at the hospital and was on life support pending arrival of the organ transplant team. Many family members had come for the ceremony. When all was in readiness, I conducted the time-of-death service, with family packed in the ICU room. The service concluded with celebration of the gift of life that would be given to many others.

The transplant team then prepared the patient for transport to surgery. As they wheeled him out, his wife and I followed, and then all the family fell in. We took the patient elevator from ICU to surgery. When we stepped out of the elevator, I was astonished. We saw the walls of the hallways all the way to surgery lined shoulder to shoulder with members of the hospital's medical and administrative staff (more than two hundred people).

The honor walk proceeded between the lines of staff

members who came to honor their fellow staff member and celebrate the gift of life he was providing to so many others.

The wife and family said their final goodbyes at the door of the surgery suite, known as "the finish line." Then I accompanied the wife and family as we reversed through the hallways, acknowledging the honor of the presence of all these staff members.

Afterward, we were told this was the first honor walk ceremony performed at this hospital and the largest attendance at an honor walk in the history of the Gift of Life organization.

Case 3.12: That's All I Want to Know

I was with the family in the family room when we were notified her husband had been pronounced. I escorted her to trauma suite 3. Their son and daughter followed.

She walked up to the bed and touched her beloved's foot, which was sticking out from under the sheet. She looked up into space and asked, "Is he with God?"

"Yes," I replied softly. "He is in God's arms and has been welcomed into eternal life."

She breathed a sigh of relief and said resolutely, "That's all I want to know."

She moved to the side of the bed and caressed her

lifelong companion's head. The son and daughter moved to the other side. I conducted a brief prayer service.

Cases 3.13: Called Back

#1. I had completed my rounds and was headed home. My phone rang as I left the parking lot. A family in ICU had requested a chaplain. I made a U-turn at the first legal opportunity and returned to hospital.

The family had made the decision to remove life support. I prayed with the patient's wife and family. Nursing staff removed life support, and I stayed with the family through the end-of-life vigil. Scriptures, prayers, committal, and comfort to the family were needed.

#2. Two hours later, I was walking toward the parking lot when my phone rang. About-face and back to the hospital. A similar scenario followed. Once again, I was where God wanted me to be.

Case 3.14: Large Family

I was informed when I arrived there was a serious case in trauma suite 3 and the patient was not expected to survive. The family was in the family room.

I passed by trauma suite 3 and could recognize the efforts of the trauma team to provide the opportunity for a miracle to save the patient.

I headed to the family room, which was packed and overflowing. The results waiting room where walk-in patients waited was empty, so I relocated the family there. They filled that room.

It was not long before the attending physician came to inform the family they had been unable to save the patient and he had expired. I prayed with the family.

Within minutes, the number of family members doubled. Fortunately, the pediatric waiting room was empty, and the additional overflow was assembled there. I held a second prayer service for the additional family members.

Cases 3.15: Timing

#1. A colleague had spent an hour with a family in the cardiac intensive care unit. The patient stabilized and appeared to be improving. He left to go to another hospital.

I was running an errand before I went to the hospital for my regular rounds when I received a call while driving (hands-free Bluetooth), asking me if I could come. I was only a few blocks from the hospital; one turn, and I was there in five minutes.

I went up to the third-floor CICU. The charge nurse said, "Your timing is perfect. He was doing fine but suddenly reversed. The family is with him."

I entered the room. A daughter was at each side of the bed, each holding a hand. I prayed and anointed the patient.

They agreed to remove life support. As I stepped to the foot of the bed, he coded. The attending nurse came in and informed the daughters he was gone.

I stepped out and spoke with the nurse. "That was amazing," she said. "You arrived at exactly the proper time." That is God's timing.

She filled me in on the details before I returned to the room to hold a brief committal service with the family.

#2. As I left the cardiac intensive care unit, code blue was announced in the oncology unit. I went straight to that unit on the fifth floor without waiting for a call.

The room was packed with doctors, nurses, and specialists. I stood in the hall and prayed with that patient's wife and son.

One of the doctors stepped out to inform the family

it did not look good. He returned in several minutes to let them know the patient had expired. Once the medical equipment had been disconnected and the nurses had left, we entered the room for an additional prayer service.

Then down to the first-floor ED for my regular rounds. My personal errands could wait.

God's plans are absolutely amazing, and His timing is beyond comprehension.

PART IV

Ecumenical:

Cases That Serve Those in Need without Discrimination

Cases 4.1: Same God

#1. I entered the room and identified myself as a member of the spiritual care team. I wear a simple wooden cross.

The patient responded he was a Muslim. He said we have the same God, but he preferred their form of prayer.

I acknowledged his position and then offered him comfort care: blanket, pillow, water, juice, coffee. He smiled appreciatively.

#2. The next week, I entered a room, and the patient identified herself as a Muslim. She also said we have the same God.

Then she said she preferred Muslim prayers but also enjoyed Christian prayer forms. I prayed to God without mentioning the Trinity.

Everybody wins.

#3. Jews are often receptive to prayer by a Christian. In this case, I focus on the God of Abraham, Isaac, and Jacob.

No problem.

Cases 4.2: Who Is Present

#1. I entered the room and engaged the young female patient in conversation. Then I asked her if she would like some prayer.

"Sure," she said with a smile.

Then she looked at her mother, who was frowning, and quickly changed her mind. "We are Jehovah's Witness, and we take care of ourselves," she said in a monotone voice.

I nodded and offered comfort care.

#2. A few weeks later, I offered prayer to another young woman. There were no others in the room.

"I am Jehovah's Witness, but I would still like prayer," she said.

Case 4.3: Buddhist

I visited a male patient who appeared to be of Western European descent. He was in good spirits. I offered prayer. He replied he was Buddhist.

He went on to say he knew quite a bit about Christianity. Then he ticked off the denominations of various family members, covering several of the better-known varieties. After that, he said he chose Buddhism because the Buddha taught service to others.

I brought him a pillow and gave it to him, saying this was to honor his faith. He responded with the largest, wide-eyed smile I have ever seen.

Case 4.4: Terminal Diagnosis

The charge nurse informed me one of the ED physicians wanted to speak with me. I went to the physicians' charting room, and she asked me to accompany her to deliver a stage 4 cancer diagnosis to a patient.

It is rare to have diagnoses in the ED, but the CAT scan was definitive, and the radiologist made the diagnosis. We headed to the patient's room.

He was the lead pastor at a large multicampus Bible church and had a doctor of theology degree.

The physician explained the pain that brought him in was from an infection secondary to a tumor that was advanced and had metastasized significantly. The course of treatment would begin immediately to cure the infection so the oncologists and surgeons could schedule treatment for the cancer.

He received the news stoically. His wife tried to be brave but was trembling.

I stood by while the attending physician answered their questions directly. She then turned to me, nodded, and excused herself. I reviewed the immediate steps with the family and reinforced the importance of following the longer-range treatment plan that would be developed.

I prayed as pastor to a pastor, reinforcing our faith and relying on the love, grace, wisdom, strength, and power of the Trinity.

The pastor glowed, and his wife began to relax.

Case 4.5: Blessing

I visited an older patient. (Remember, I am older, so I can say that with respect.) I prayed for God's healing grace for him, comfort to family and friends, and guidance to the medical team.

He said he was a retired minister and understood the importance of my ministry. He took my hand and prayed for me, thanking God for my service.

Next, he placed his hand on my heart and blessed me. Then he said quite sincerely, "Now get going. There are lots of patients out there who need you."

Case 4.6: Pastor to Pastor

I greeted the patient with my usual introduction, "Hi, my name is Tom. I am a member of the spiritual care team."

The patient quickly responded, "I am a pastor."

He served an established independent Bible church in the area. We had an old-fashioned "come to Jesus" prayer session.

Case 4.7: Atheist

I entered the room and saw a male patient. His wife was sitting at his bedside. I introduced myself and offered prayer.

"I don't believe," the man said politely, "but my wife might like it." He gritted his teeth.

I prayed briefly for comfort and healing, for family

and friends, and for all those who provide service to others.

When I finished, his wife was beaming.

I looked at him. He had this pleasant look of amazement on his face. No attempt to convert him, only to care for him and let him know others did too.

Case 4.8: Chaplain's Chaplain

A beaming face greeted me. I introduced myself, and the patient responded he was a chaplain and was pleased to see another show up without being called.

He was an ecumenical chaplain. In fact, he stated he would not pastor a church, as that was too narrow a ministry.

We prayed for each other. He was a bright spot in my day, and I in his. Mutual care was an uplifting experience for both of us.

When it was time to leave, he said he better understood the value and power of a spiritual care visit.

Case 4.9: Coverage

The call came before dawn. A teenage trauma patient did not make it. The family asked for a chaplain to give

Catholic last rites (sacrament of healing). The on-call priest designated by the dioceses was not available. His backup was undergoing chemotherapy and could not come. The family could not reach their parish priest.

I headed to the hospital to be with the family for spiritual comfort. While on the way, friends of the family were able to reach a priest who could come. I stayed with the family until he arrived.

Cases 4.10: Double, Double

#1. There was a large group of family in the family room—husband, sister, children, and nieces and nephews. The patient was on life support, and one family member at a time rotated to sit with her. I prayed for the patient, her family, and the medical team. The family was in good spirits. I brought coffee to the husband and sister.

A gentleman was seated near the door. As I turned to leave, he reached out, shook my hand, and said he was a pastor also. His face was glowing with warmth and appreciation that a stranger came to pray for and provide comfort care to members of his flock.

#2. Three patient visits later, I entered a room with an elderly couple (remember, I can say elderly because I am elderly). The wife was the patient. Her husband was seated in a chair at her bedside, with his hands folded on top of his cane.

The patient was in some pain. She was tense and showed signs of foreboding. As I prayed for her, her family, and the medical team, I could see the tenseness relax and a sense of hope begin to show.

When I finished, the husband asked me to come to his side of the bed so he could shake the hand of a fellow servant of Christ. He was a retired pastor.

Two grateful pastors in one day—a double, double.

Postscript: Thee days later, I was greeted with "Hi, Dr. Tom!" as I entered the hospital. Seated in the lobby were the husband and two daughters of the large family I had prayed with in Case 4.10 #1. They said the patient had recovered, was in ICU, and would be going home that day.

I rarely get closure, but God sent another message to me that day: "Well done, good and faithful conduit."

Case 4.11: I Wish

I visited a patient and his wife. He was in a hall bed, as all the ED rooms were occupied. He had the edge of a pillowcase covering his forehead and eyes to shade the bright light. He peered out from under as I prayed for him, smiled slightly, and covered his eyes again.

Sometime later, I was completing my rounds, visiting the last few rooms on the unit. As I entered one, the patient said, "We saw you in the hall."

I recognized the wife from the earlier hall visit. I told them I was glad we were able to get them moved into a room. The patient grumbled it was not much of a room, but it was more restful.

Then he asked my church. I told him I worshiped at a Christian church but that I ministered to all. He replied, "I wish I could be a Christian." His wife nodded.

As we talked, the patient explained two views of Christianity he had. The first was why limit God by definition. I could understand that view and suggested focusing on Christ as God's gift to all. He softened.

Then he expressed confusion from the proliferation of denominations, some professing their belief was the only correct belief in Christ. I could understand this too and suggested each person develop a personal relationship with Christ.

We ended with mutual agreement that God was in charge and we could rely on that.

Case 4.12: International

Four chaplains from Brazil came to the US for more training. They were the coordinators for eighty volunteer chaplains. One was bilingual and was the translator. The others spoke Portuguese and little English. I was asked to host a portion of their visit and take them on a tour of my hospital.

Their first comment was their emergency rooms were open, with lots of beds, and they were impressed with private rooms in our ED, with hall beds for overflow. I would ask a patient if it was OK if they sat in on a visit before inviting them to join me in a room. We also walked through other units of the hospital.

While on the tour, I received a call that a patient recovering from cardiac surgery requested a visit. My Brazilian guests accompanied me to the cardiac postsurgery unit. I prayed for the patient, and while we were visiting, she said she was from Brazil. Immediately the Brazilian chaplains began to visit with her in Portuguese. God's timing is amazing.

As my new friends and colleagues were leaving, they asked for a copy of a couple of my prayers. I pray extemporaneously, but I made a mental note of what they were asking. I wrote the prayers from my memory and used a language translator to provide a copy in Portuguese. I emailed both the English and Portuguese versions to them.

Case 4.13: Thanks for Answering

I entered the room and saw what appeared to be a distraught female patient. I introduced myself and asked if she would care for prayer. She hesitated and then said, "I guess so."

As I prayed, she relaxed. She smiled when I finished. I asked if she needed anything. She said her daughter was coming and would get her some ice for her soda. I replied she did not have to wait and returned with a cup of ice.

She said, "That was a beautiful prayer. Do you have a church?"

I replied, "I attend a church, but I'm a volunteer chaplain."

She said she attended a Missionary Baptist church and inquired why I came to her room.

I replied, "God sends me little messages."

She smiled again and said, "Thanks for answering."

Case 4.14: Betrayal or Faith

When I finished praying for the female patient, she held onto my hand and squeezed it. "Thank you," she whispered. "That is what I needed to hear."

She then explained she was a member of a denomination that told her she needed to pray harder for healing, not go to the hospital. She felt she had betrayed her church by being in the ED, that her faith was not strong enough to heal her.

In my prayer, I had asked for God to continue to guide the medical team. This had helped her understand God was doing the healing by using some of His servants.

In further discussions, we concluded that God works through others, but He oversees the result. The efforts of His skilled servants are His way of healing.

I suggested she was demonstrating her faith by allowing those God had trained to assist with her healing. When the best efforts of these knowledgeable workers are insufficient, God provides healing beyond their skills or calls us home.

The tension drained from her body. She relaxed and was smiling when the attending physician came into the room. He reached out to shake my hand and gave me a warm smile.

Cases 4.15: Taking Service to Those in Need

When I began my ED visitation rounds on Ash Wednesday, my phone started to fill with text requests for ashes from patients elsewhere in the hospital who could not go to the chapel during the hour when a local Catholic priest and a local Protestant minister imposed ashes. Among these were the open-heart surgery patient in cardiac recovery ICU and her family, the brand-new mother and father in postpartum, the heart patient and his family in CICU, and the critically ill patient and her family in ICU.

Upon returning to the ED, I passed by the associate medical director, who was studying a patient chart. She greeted me and said they were so busy she could not get away to go to the chapel.

When I told her I had ashes, she exclaimed, "Rock on!" stopped what she was doing, and stood to receive ashes. Later, as we passed in the hall, she said, "Thanks so much."

Nurses, aides, and technicians would stop as we passed in the hall and ask for ashes.

I took a break for a quick lunch. As I entered the cafeteria, the nursing education director was leaving. She nodded to me and remarked, "We've been too busy today."

I told her I had ashes. She stopped and simply said, "Please." Immediately, three other nurses lined up to receive ashes.

This ministry meets people where they are, without regard to who or what they are.

Case 4.16: Old-Timers

Most of the patients and families I serve are strangers. One notable exception was the day I stepped into a patient room in the ED and saw a friend lying on the bed.

We had been to many meetings together for a non-church-related spiritual fellowship I had been active in for almost four decades. The patient had participated for more than three decades. As the patient finished explaining why he was in the ED, a common friend who also had more than three decades of activity in that same spiritual fellowship popped in.

There we were, more than a century of service in this outstanding spiritual fellowship. We had an old-timers meeting. We recalled our service to one another and to countless others over those many years. It was healing and invigorating for all of us.

He was in good spirits when he was admitted to ICU. I continued to visit this friend over the next few weeks as he weakened and his condition became more severe. Many of our mutual friends came to visit him.

I was able to be with his family when they made the final decision to remove life support.

Our time of joyous remembrances was a comfort to the patient and to me.

PART V

Care and Comfort:

Cases That Combine Compassion with Spiritual Care

Case 5.1: Nobody Has Come

I entered the room where an older woman patient was lying very still. An older man was seated to the left. He was apparently her husband. He had a cane between his knees. A middle-aged man and woman were standing to the right. Apparently, they were children or a child and spouse.

One of the children said, "Who is this?"

"He's in the wrong room," the husband retorted. There was an edge in his voice.

I didn't respond but went to the bedside and looked down at the patient. Since she was either sound asleep or in some sort of coma, I turned back to the husband. I introduced myself, asked her name, and asked if we could have some prayer for her.

The husband responded guardedly. I prayed for her, her family, and the medical team. As I turned to leave, the husband stood up. He was five or six inches taller than me (and I am six feet tall). He reached out and took my hand with a grip so strong it was close to leaving a bruise.

With a bright, warm smile, he said, "The children and I pray for her every morning. She has been sick for seven years. You are the first person who has come to pray for her." His eyes were glistening.

I went to greet the children, who had a pleasant look of surprise and appreciation on their faces. They declined any refreshments, but the husband took a cup of coffee.

Several minutes later, I saw the husband in the hall. When he saw me, his face lit. It was the light of Christ shining back at me.

Case 5.2: Obnoxious

I was passing by the nursing station and heard a nurse complaining to the charge nurse that her patient was impossible, uncooperative, restive, and obnoxious. She asked to have another nurse assigned to this disagreeable patient.

The charge nurse, said, "Send Dr. Tom in. He'll give him a sandwich and a prayer." I stopped and turned to the charge nurse, who smiled and nodded at me.

I looked in the room and saw a young man sitting on the edge of the bed, rigid as a board, so I went one better. I brought him a prayer, a sandwich, and a can of Sprite.

He had never been in a hospital and had no idea what to expect. He was scared. Christ's love was demonstrated through kindness.

The patient relaxed, leaned back on the bed, and cooperated fully with the nurse he had resisted.

Case 5.3: Rookie Mistake

After prayer, I offered something to drink for the patient. He asked for apple juice. I went to the patient nutrition room, opened an individual-size container of apple juice, and poured it in a clear plastic cup.

As I was walking back to the patient's room, the head of security for the unit passed going the other way. He smiled and remarked, "I hope that is apple juice."

There I was carrying amber liquid in a clear drinking

glass. Samples of the same color liquid are taken in sealed containers to the lab for analysis. Whoops. I pour apple juice into an opaque Styrofoam cup now.

Case 5.4: A Repeater

As I entered the emergency department, an aide said, "Room 26 is asking for you."

As I passed the nurse's station, one of the clerks said, "Room 26 wanted to know if you would be in today before she would even register."

I went to room 26. I had visited with the female patient three months prior. She was back for medical care for a different illness. Spiritual care was so important to her; she wanted assurance it would be available on this visit.

Christ's impressions are lasting.

Case 5.5: Reviving Spiritual Care Service

The patient was a young man, resting well despite being a little apprehensive. The attending nurse was entering charting information into the computer terminal. I used that opportunity to pray with the patient. The nurse paused and listened prayerfully.

As I was leaving, the patient said to the nurse, "You don't see that much anymore."

"Oh, we have it here," the nurse responded proudly.

Case 5.6: Parental Comfort

The call came from a labor and delivery nurse. She relayed that the case was an eighteen-week fetal demise. The mother wanted it blessed.

I responded and blessed the stillborn fetus. Then I spent some time comforting the mother and father.

I went to the chapel for my own care. I had responded to the need instinctually and now wondered if I had performed a service not recognized by some churches.

The answer came before I could even begin to meditate. I heard through my conscience, "Do not worry. I sanctioned this. Well done."

Later, I double-checked with a pastor friend, who encouraged me to continue to follow that instinct.

Case 5.7: Administrative Feedback

I was heading toward the main entrance at the end of a busy day in the ED. The associate director of nursing for the entire hospital was walking the other direction.

She stopped, turned to me, and said, "I was hoping to find you today. I have a message from my mother. You prayed for her in the ED Monday. She could not remember your name, but I knew it was you. She asked me to thank you for your visit and to be sure to tell you how much it meant to her."

That was a paycheck from God, more valuable than pure gold.

Case 5.8: Calm

Patients with mental illness are placed on psychiatric hold until a commitment decision can be made. One such case was severely agitated. The medical staff could not calm her and were considering having to place her in restraints. The head security officer called me over and asked me to visit her.

I went into the room, where I saw the patient writhing and thrashing her arms and legs. Her boyfriend was trying to hold her. Staff was trying to soothe her but ended up only able to keep her from flipping off the bed. She was not fighting them off, but she still was not calming down.

I addressed her by name. She looked up at me with a blank stare and continued to squirm.

I placed my hand on her forehead and began to speak slowly. She stopped squirming and lay still.

I prayed for peace of mind and a quiet spirit for her. It was a brief prayer. She closed her eyes, lay still, and began to breathe slowly and deeply. She was asleep.

I tiptoed out of the room. The security officer followed me out. He shook my hand. "You do wonders for these folks," he said.

I replied, "Glad I could help." She was frightened, whether in a psychotic break or not. A calm voice from an older person assured her she would be fine.

Case 5.9: Healing

I entered the room and saw an elderly gentleman lying on the bed. His wife was seated beside him. When she looked up and saw me, she wailed, "Oh no, he is dying!"

"No, ma'am," I replied quickly. "I came to pray for healing."

She relaxed and said, "Oh, the only time I ever see a minister in the hospital is when someone is dying."

I did not respond to her observation, because it is true. Instead, I offered prayer for healing, comfort to family, and guidance to the medical team to restore health. Then I offered her a cup of coffee.

When I returned with her coffee, she was smiling. "He's feeling better already," she said.

I looked at the patient, and he winked at me. She was the one who was feeling better. He was in good spirits because he was not worrying about her worrying about him.

Case 5.10: Encore

Nine months after Case 1.1, I entered a patient's room. The family member looked up and burst into a grin. "It's you!" she exclaimed. "I have to give you a hug."

She jumped up and came straight to me for a big hug.

Then she turned to the patient and told her, "He was the only one there the day of the high school shooting. There were people all over the place. Finally, some pastors came, but this is the hospital chaplain who took care of all of us."

We reminisced about the trauma of the school shooting. She was a nursing instructor at a local college and was in the hospital with her students. She was able to give directions to restrooms, the cafeteria, and the gift shop, but that was about all she could do, she remembered.

I prayed with the patient, who had become calm and

relaxed as she heard of the extra effort the entire staff extended to all patients.

When I excused myself in a few minutes, I had this warm feeling. It was a "Well done" from God, a delayed paycheck.

Cases 5.11: Uno, Duo, Tres

I was called to attend a death on the medical surgical unit. As I entered the unit, a nurse intercepted me and took me to the family room. There I found the adult son, his girlfriend, and three of his close friends.

The son was distraught, crying as he said, "I don't want to lose both parents in two days."

The backstory began to unfold. His mother was the patient in the hospital. She had a seizure two days ago, so he was frightened for her health. His father took his mother to the hospital, where she was stabilized, and then went home for the night. The son came the next morning to pick up his father and go to the hospital, but he found his father dead on the floor from an apparent heart attack. He spent the day with EMS, police, and the coroner. Then he was afraid to tell his mother for fear of another seizure.

The girlfriend then disclosed that the son also had

heart trouble and had just changed heart medication. She was fearful of the strain on him.

Suddenly, there were three cases in one. The mother was under medical care, so she became #3. The father was at the coroner and became #2. The son was in immediate distress and became #1.

I was able to get the son to talk about all the events calmly. With the support of his girlfriend and his three close friends, we were able to maintain his composure. Then we had prayer for the father and committed him to God's eternal care. Next, we faced the challenge of telling the mother her husband had died the day before.

Nursing staff were standing by with the crisis cart. I remained outside, as seeing a chaplain unannounced would have shocked the mother. The son and his girlfriend were able to explain all that had happened, and I was then called in.

The mother's first reaction was that this was backward; she was to go first, not her husband. Counseling and prayer for comfort and healing were able to provide a reasonable stability so the crisis cart could be released.

The single case doubled, then tripled, and all were resolved by God's grace.

Case 5.12: Disturbed

I had just arrived on the unit and was restocking the blanket warmer. An aide stopped me and asked, "Can you visit with the patient in 19? She asked for the chaplain." I told her I would be there just as soon as I finished.

The aide was assigned to sit with the patient, who was on a psychiatric watch. I pulled the physician's stool over and sat beside her bed. She was huddled in a ball under a blanket but peered out. I told her I understood she wanted to talk, and she nodded.

"What brings you to our august institution?" I asked.

"I did some things that were not appropriate," was her guarded reply, but she was able to look directly at me.

I reached out and took her hands, which were peeking out from under the blanket. There was no need for details, only to offer assurances she was in the right place doing the right things now. I prayed for guidance and skilled care and for openness to receive the help she needed.

She relaxed and uncoiled from the ball but remained in a fetal position. I talked with her some more. She nodded and made some brief replies, acknowledging that she was listening.

I assured her what she had done was history and that she would be fine and not need to repeat that behavior. She flexed her legs for the first time and lifted her head off the bed and onto the pillow.

She had a pleasant smile when I left.

Case 5.13: Needed

As I stepped into trauma suite 3 in the ED, I saw a distraught mother holding her young baby. Nursing staff were quickly administering treatment as she cradled her critically ill infant. There is a trauma room in the pediatrics section of the ED, but the more severe cases are treated in one of the major trauma suites in the larger, full-service ED section.

She looked up at me and said, "You prayed for us in NICU last month. We need you even more now." I recognized her and remembered her twins. The other twin was at home with the father.

I prayed without interfering with the nurses as they feverishly administered treatment. They smiled and nodded when I finished.

The mother relaxed as I handed her a Kleenex.

Case 5.14: Blanket Vendor,
a.k.a. Comfort Care

The man was standing in the hall outside the door while the medical staff performed a procedure on his wife. As I walked up, he said, "We know you. You have the most important job here. You give out the warm blankets." He went on to explain his wife had been a patient in the ED three months before for a less severe condition and how much they appreciated the care, especially the warm blankets.

The same reaction is received for a pillow. I can see the tension relieved in the neck and shoulders when I place a fresh pillow under the patient's head (when appropriate). Often, I pat them gently and say, "See? We can do some things right." When they smile, fear and apprehension are lessened.

Comfort care is as important as spiritual care.

Epilogue

After my first month serving in the emergency department, I was asked to be the spiritual care advisor to the NICU quality of care team and make rounds in the NICU whenever I could. Then a month later, I was asked to take calls for spiritual care throughout the hospital. As I lived only fifteen minutes from the hospital, I agreed to take calls 24-7 (twenty-four hours a day, seven days a week).

In three years, I visited seventeen thousand individuals. Of these, 8,500 were patients, 7,500 were family members and close friends of a patient, and 1,000 were staff. Less than 1 percent were repeat visits.

After three years of making regular rounds in the emergency department, making occasional rounds in NICU, and responding to calls throughout the hospital, all chaplains, including me, were furloughed due to the COVID-19 pandemic. Chaplains had community contacts in addition to hospital contacts, and the risk of carrying the virus from one to the other was too high.

While furloughed, I turned my attention to Zoom virtual sessions with both new and longtime members of a spiritual fellowship I had been active in for almost four decades. That is the spiritual fellowship mentioned in Case 4.16: Old Timers.

Seven months later, I was the first chaplain allowed to return to service under strict rules to protect both my health and that of the patients and staff. Only single visits were allowed, meaning there would be limited family interaction, but patients and staff still needed spiritual care. I reported to administration to be reoriented. I submitted my current vaccination documents and was cleared to make rounds immediately.

I was greeted with cheers when I entered the emergency department. Nurses were applauding and waving. Eyes were wide and smiling over masks. "Welcome back! We missed you," was repeated multiple times. When I passed by the ED manager's office, she exclaimed, "Dr. Tom, you're back! We sure need you." Nurses lined up for prayers. Doctors stopped in the hall to say, "Good to see you! You were missed."

This conduit was home. My service continues …

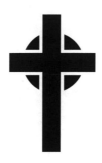

Printed in the United States
by Baker & Taylor Publisher Services